PROLOGUE

This book is dedicated to all the children, teens, adults, and parents who have experienced themselves or loved ones who have given up all hope and the will to live. My prayer is that this rainbow journey will provide a flicker of hope and cause for reflection to guide one to better days.

Prolonged sadness may lead to depression. If you or someone you know is suffering from depression, please seek professional help.

If you are having thoughts of suicide, call or text 988 to reach the National Suicide Prevention Lifeline or go to SpeakingOfSuicide.com/resources for a list of additional resources.

Note: Any resources mentioned are not promoted or sponsored by the author but are simply suggested references for your use.

To my two shining stars – always - CHASE and DREW.

To my inspiration Eric T.

In loving memory of my mom and dad – and my big sister, Janet, who always loved books.

Chase's Story

Chase is my daughter. This is for her and all the young women who struggle silently with depression and anxiety, who may not have the support required to have the normal life they so desperately desire.

Chase's depression and anxiety didn't appear until she left for college. Near the end of her sophomore semester, she had to take a leave of absence.

The depression and anxiety were overwhelming, and her life began to spiral out of control. She was unable to push through anymore. This forced her to seek professional help. It was during this time that she was diagnosed and decided to take the time needed to focus on her mental health.

Chase spent a year and a half with multiple therapists, psychiatrists, day programs, and a two-month residential program. Since she stepped away from school, she has been fighting for a quality of life most of us take for granted.

Along this healing journey, she discovered that she loves music. She transferred from an elite tech school that wasn't where she really wanted to be, to a university with a music program that fit her career goals.

With the coping tools and a consistent support system, Chase now lives on her own and is back in school with a 3.7 GPA and three semesters to complete her music degree.

She still struggles with getting out of bed some mornings and dealing with moments of great sadness. She approaches life one day at a time. The combination of the coping tools learned in therapy, family, friends, therapists, and her university's support staff have enabled her to navigate her challenges.

I pray for the parents and students who are dealing with mental health challenges. I encourage them to get help if needed. It's okay to not always be okay.

I often share with Chase that she is a beacon of light and that even the sun doesn't shine with the same brightness each day, but it always shows up providing whatever it is able to provide.

I say to her...Thank you! Shine on! ♥

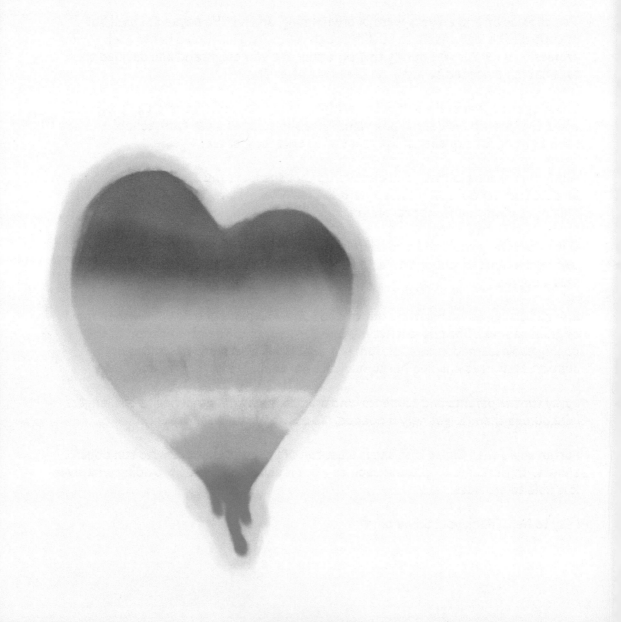

This story journal
belongs to :

_____

PRESSURE! SO MUCH PRESSURE! Grades, "friends" not being friends, my "significant other" not so significant after all, hating my major, living on my own with bills. I thought "adulting" would be fun! I couldn't wait to leave home and be in college hanging out with new friends, doing what I want when I want, cool parties, and no curfews. At least, that's how I imagined life to be after graduating high school. Sigh.

I'm Indigo. I grew up in a small town in Kentucky with my younger sister, Violet, my parents, and our little fluffy, one-eyed Yorkie, Gizmo. For the most part, I had a pretty decent childhood. I've always been a kid my parents could be proud of, and a good role model for my little sister, Violet. However, it was around my junior year in high school that the proverbial sh** hit the fan.

Suddenly, I was just burnt out from everything I once enjoyed doing – the rigorous schoolwork, volleyball, president of the National "Super-Smart Students" Club, honors orchestra. Everything became overwhelming including the competitive and stressful process of applying for colleges. It was like my life just came to a complete stop. I started avoiding going to class, volleyball practice, and orchestra rehearsals. It was getting difficult just to get out of bed most days. It felt like the weight of the world was on my shoulders. As my mother would say, "What in the heebee-jeebee is going on?"

My parents were worried, and I was terrified. Thankfully, my parents took immediate action by talking to the school principal and counselors and getting me into therapy to seek help. I was diagnosed

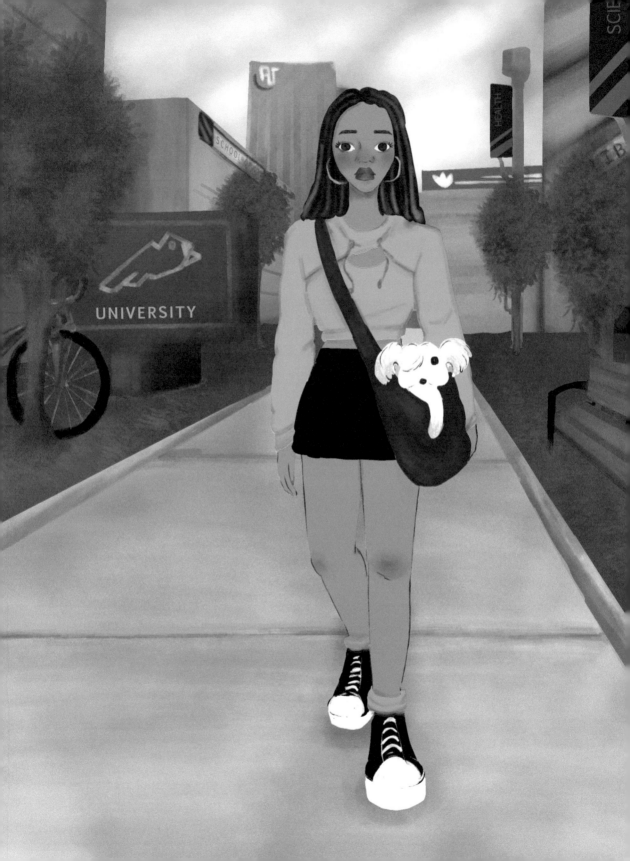

with depression and anxiety and spent some intensive time in therapy. Over time I had a support system in place with school, friends, and family, and I was taught coping tools to manage my depressive symptoms and return to my normal life. I was also able to register our dog, Gizmo, as an emotional support animal (ESA) to help with my sadness and anxiety.

I'm now a sophomore, with my little dog Gizmo, attending a major university in the cool city of Atlanta. As I walk across the campus, the skies are cloudy and gray with the promise of rain to come. I think about how much I love it here, living on my own, relishing the whole university experience, and enjoying the hustle and bustle of urban life. However, lately, all I've been feeling is PRESSURE, and it's really bogging me down. Everything around me just seems off and out of place. I've learned from therapy that there are triggers that can affect my depression and anxiety, and I need to peel away the onion and figure out what is going on because now I'm worried about everything... my grades, the "adulting", my life. I'm even starting to question if my friends are really my friends, and if I'm in the right major.

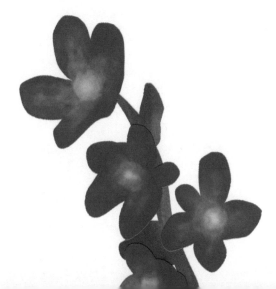

I'm majoring in pre-med because I've always been good in chemistry and my parents heavily prompted me to pursue medicine. While it would be cool to be a doctor, it's not really what I love or want to be. I'm actually a low-key gamer and want to design video games. I love the coding, the visualizations, the creativity. I feel amazing just thinking about it!

I continue walking through the campus and let the thoughts flow. It begins to rain, and I pull out my umbrella to cover Gizmo and me. As I wallow lost in my thoughts, the rain abruptly ends and lo and behold, I notice a beautiful, wavy rainbow graphic up ahead! There it flows in a wondrous spectrum of red, orange, yellow, green, blue, indigo, and violet, or as we know it, ROY G BIV.

I begin to imagine the colors as a representation of my life, my ups and downs, the triggers that are causing my mental disruption at this moment.

My mind wanders as I imagine riding the rainbow...

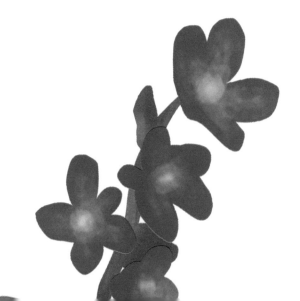

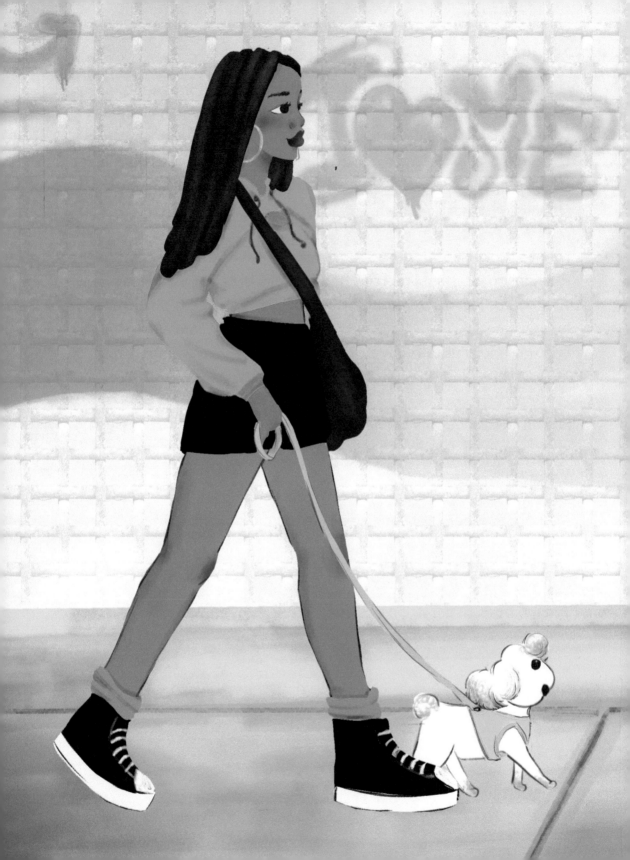

R is for REALITY

WELCOME TO THE REAL WORLD.
You are "adulting" and this new reality can be very daunting and stressful.

STOP. Be still. Count to 10 and breathe. The reality is that you have evolved from a "perfect child" into "an imperfect teen/young adult". It's ok not to be perfect.

ACTION!
Think about the causes or triggers that made you feel anxious.

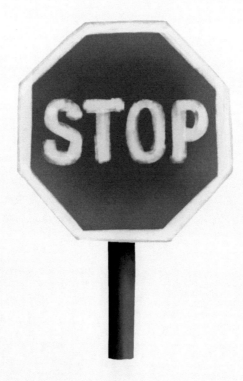

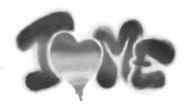

What makes you feel overwhelmed?

_____

_____

_____

_____

_____

_____

_____

_____

_____

_____

_____

_____

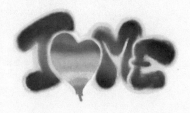

_____

_____

_____

_____

_____

_____

_____

_____

_____

_____

_____

_____

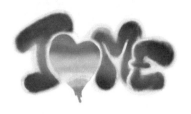

_____

_____

_____

_____

_____

_____

_____

_____

_____

_____

_____

_____

_____

_____

_____

O is for OWN IT

OWN IT. PEEL AWAY the blame until you get to the sweet spot of accountability and control.

ACTION!
Think about an orange. The outside peeling doesn't taste good, but it protects the juicy, tasty, sweet inside of the orange. Now that you know how to be accountable for your actions, think about what improvements you can make.

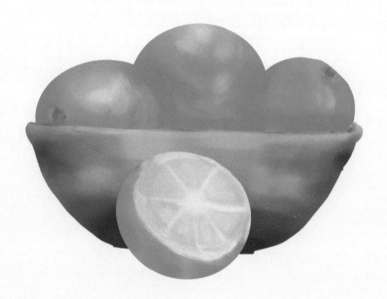

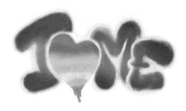

What can you do to "own" both the good and the challenging moments?

_____

_____

_____

_____

_____

_____

_____

_____

_____

_____

_____

_____

_____

_____

_____

_____

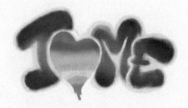

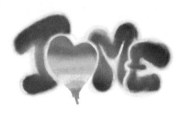

Y is for You

TAKE CARE OF YOU.
Get some sun, feel the warmth, see the light, and let it soothe you. **Celebrate your own light!**

ACTION!
Sit outside in the warmth of the sun and relax, be present, let your mind wander. Enjoy You.

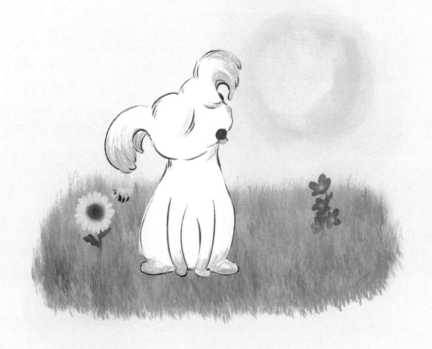

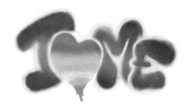

What may others see in you that you might not see in yourself?

_____

_____

_____

_____

_____

_____

_____

_____

_____

_____

_____

_____

_____

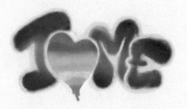

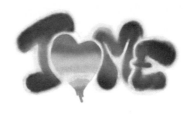

_____

_____

_____

_____

_____

_____

_____

_____

_____

_____

_____

_____

_____

_____

_____

_____

G is for GROUNDED

BE GROUNDED IN NATURE.
Embrace the nature around you.

ACTION!
Take your shoes off and walk in the grass. Feel the nature surrounding you and let it soothe you.

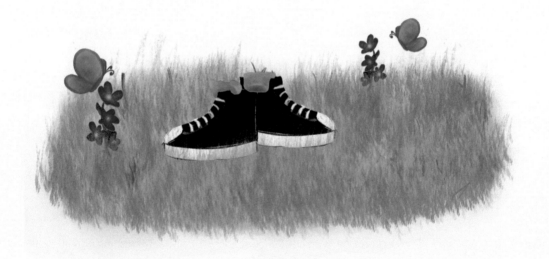

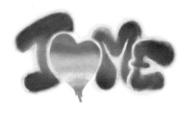

What is your favorite season and what do you enjoy doing in nature during that time?

_____

_____

_____

_____

_____

_____

_____

_____

_____

_____

_____

_____

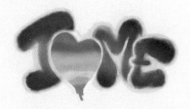

_____

_____

_____

_____

_____

_____

_____

_____

_____

_____

_____

_____

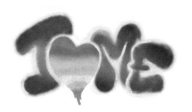

B is for BLAH

FEELING BLAH IS OK.
Some days are filled with depression, anxiety and feeling blue. It's ok not to be ok.

ACTION!
Allow yourself to feel and let go. Even have a good cry.

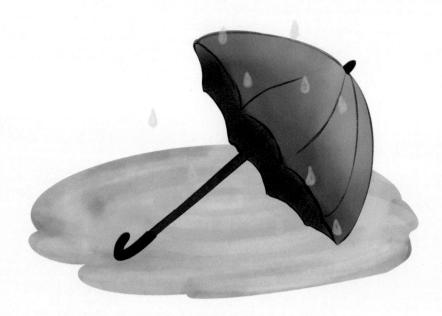

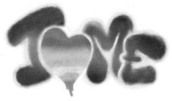

How do you feel before you cry? How do you feel after you cry? What coping tools do you use to pull you out of depressive thoughts and anxiety (eg. listening to music, meditating, drawing)?

_____

_____

_____

_____

_____

_____

_____

_____

_____

_____

_____

_____

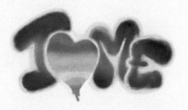

_____

_____

_____

_____

_____

_____

_____

_____

_____

_____

_____

_____

_____

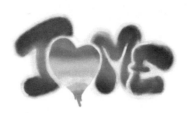

I is for INSIGHT

WHO AM I? INDIGO MEANS WISDOM AND AWARENESS.
Seek clarity and truth. Be honest with yourself and others.

LIVE YOUR LIFE the way you want to live.

ACTION!
Look into a mirror. Really look at yourself and think about who you are and the things you enjoy doing – what makes you smile. Think about what you are passionate about – what makes your heart beat a little faster with joy and anticipation.

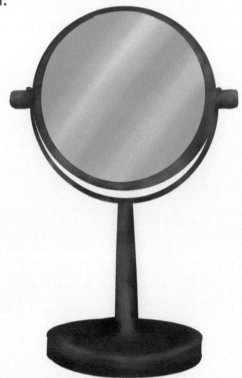

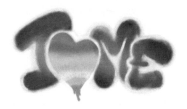

What are some of your traits that are unique to you? Are you doing what you really enjoy or what others are expecting of you? What are you doing for you vs. What are you doing for others?

_____

_____

_____

_____

_____

_____

_____

_____

_____

_____

_____

_____

_____

_____

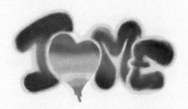

_____

_____

_____

_____

_____

_____

_____

_____

_____

_____

_____

_____

_____

_____

_____

_____

_____

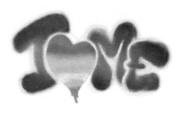

_____

_____

_____

_____

_____

_____

_____

_____

_____

_____

_____

_____

_____

_____

V is for VIBRANT

Think of a flower or plant with **VIBRANT COLORS.**
EMBRACE THE BEAUTY AND BE GRATEFUL for such
wonders in the world.

ACTION!
Describe your favorite flower or plant in detail and what
you like about it (color, scent...).

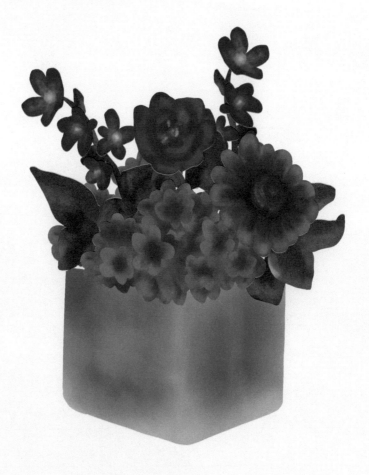

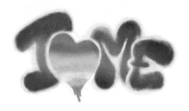

What are you most grateful for?

_____

_____

_____

_____

_____

_____

_____

_____

_____

_____

_____

_____

_____

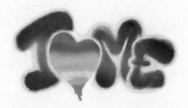

_____

_____

_____

_____

_____

_____

_____

_____

_____

_____

_____

_____

_____

_____

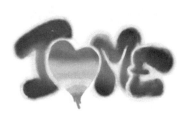

_____

_____

_____

_____

_____

_____

_____

_____

_____

_____

_____

_____

_____

_____

Riding the rainbow was an incredible experience that taught me that I am valuable and that I LOVE myself.

It is a journey through a wave of colors that have uplifted me.

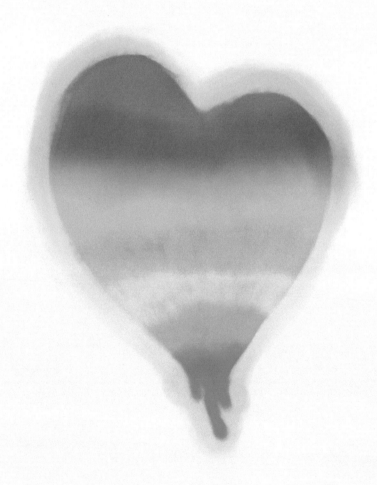

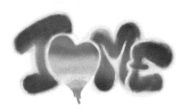

What do you LOVE about yourself?

_____

_____

_____

_____

_____

_____

_____

_____

_____

_____

_____

_____

_____

_____

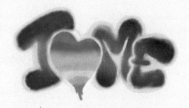

_____

_____

_____

_____

_____

_____

_____

_____

_____

_____

_____

_____

_____

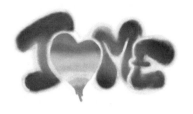

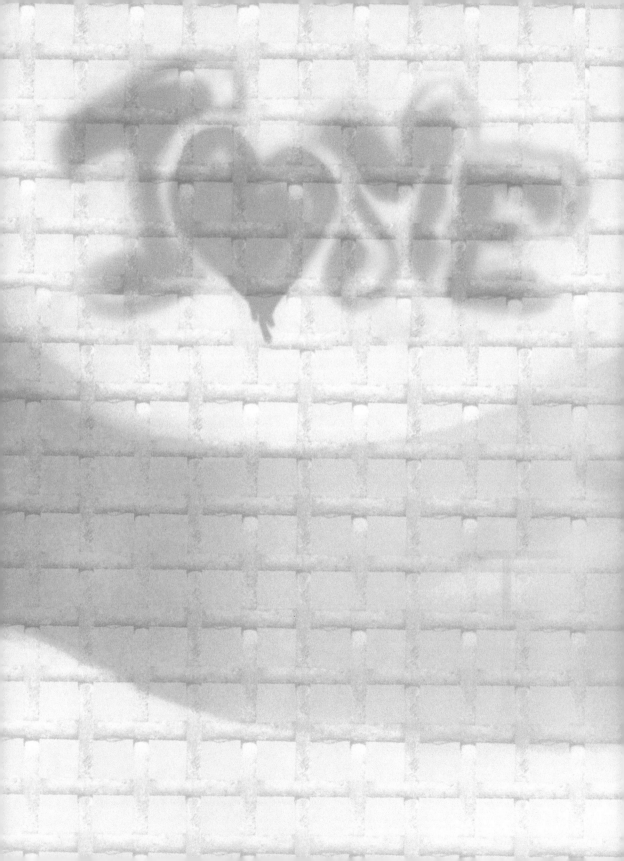

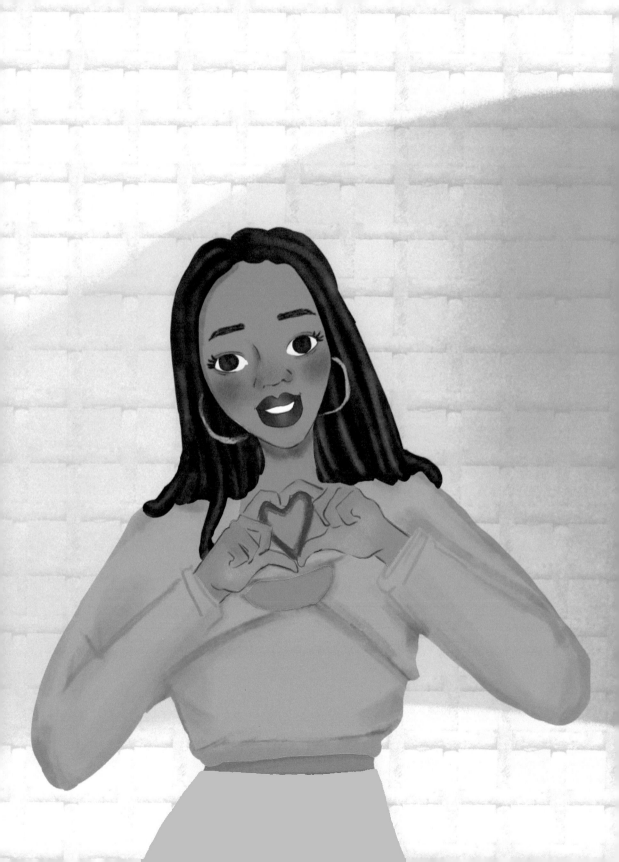

My hopes,
My thoughts,
My dreams

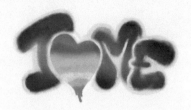

_____

_____

_____

_____

_____

_____

_____

_____

_____

_____

_____

_____

_____

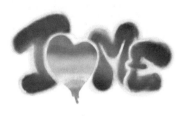

_____

_____

_____

_____

_____

_____

_____

_____

_____

_____

_____

_____

_____

_____

_____

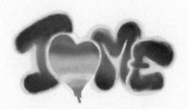

_____

_____

_____

_____

_____

_____

_____

_____

_____

_____

_____

_____

_____

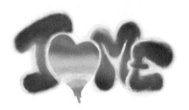

_____

_____

_____

_____

_____

_____

_____

_____

_____

_____

_____

_____

_____

_____

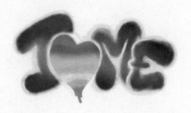

_____

_____

_____

_____

_____

_____

_____

_____

_____

_____

_____

_____

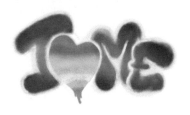

_____

_____

_____

_____

_____

_____

_____

_____

_____

_____

_____

_____

_____

_____

_____

_____

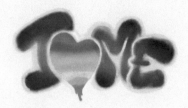

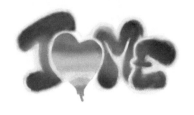

_____

_____

_____

_____

_____

_____

_____

_____

_____

_____

_____

_____

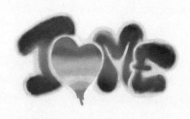

_____

_____

_____

_____

_____

_____

_____

_____

_____

_____

_____

_____

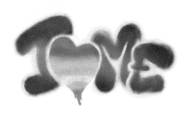

_____

_____

_____

_____

_____

_____

_____

_____

_____

_____

_____

_____

_____

_____

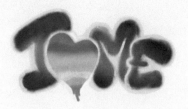

_____

_____

_____

_____

_____

_____

_____

_____

_____

_____

_____

_____

_____

_____

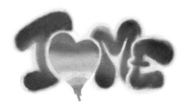

_____

_____

_____

_____

_____

_____

_____

_____

_____

_____

_____

_____

_____

_____

_____

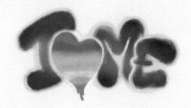

_____

_____

_____

_____

_____

_____

_____

_____

_____

_____

_____

_____

_____

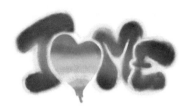

_____

_____

_____

_____

_____

_____

_____

_____

_____

_____

_____

_____

_____

_____

_____

_____

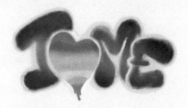

_____

_____

_____

_____

_____

_____

_____

_____

_____

_____

_____

_____

_____

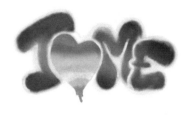

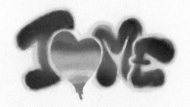

_____

_____

_____

_____

_____

_____

_____

_____

_____

_____

_____

_____

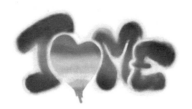

_____

_____

_____

_____

_____

_____

_____

_____

_____

_____

_____

_____

_____

_____

_____

_____

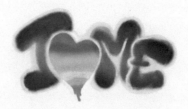

_____

_____

_____

_____

_____

_____

_____

_____

_____

_____

_____

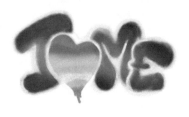

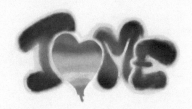

_____

_____

_____

_____

_____

_____

_____

_____

_____

_____

_____

_____

_____

_____

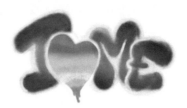

_____

_____

_____

_____

_____

_____

_____

_____

_____

_____

_____

_____

_____

_____

_____

_____

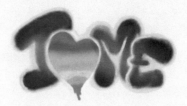

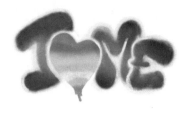

_____

_____

_____

_____

_____

_____

_____

_____

_____

_____

_____

_____

_____

_____

_____

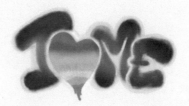

_____

_____

_____

_____

_____

_____

_____

_____

_____

_____

_____

_____

_____

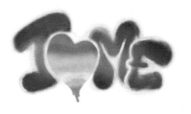

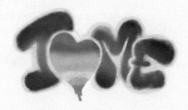

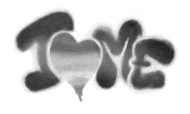

_____

_____

_____

_____

_____

_____

_____

_____

_____

_____

_____

_____

_____

_____

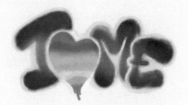

_____

_____

_____

_____

_____

_____

_____

_____

_____

_____

_____

_____

_____

_____

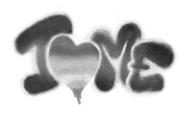

_____

_____

_____

_____

_____

_____

_____

_____

_____

_____

_____

_____

_____

_____

_____

_____

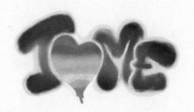

_____

_____

_____

_____

_____

_____

_____

_____

_____

_____

_____

_____

_____

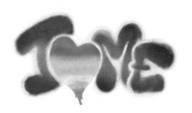

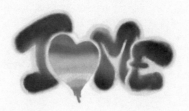

_____

_____

_____

_____

_____

_____

_____

_____

_____

_____

_____

_____

_____

_____

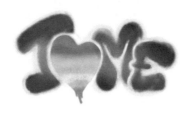

_____

_____

_____

_____

_____

_____

_____

_____

_____

_____

_____

_____

_____

_____

_____

_____

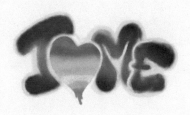

_____

_____

_____

_____

_____

_____

_____

_____

_____

_____

_____

_____

_____

_____

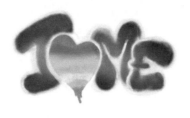

_____

_____

_____

_____

_____

_____

_____

_____

_____

_____

_____

_____

_____

_____

_____

_____

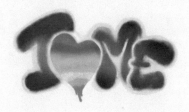

_____

_____

_____

_____

_____

_____

_____

_____

_____

_____

_____

_____

_____

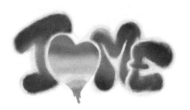

_____

_____

_____

_____

_____

_____

_____

_____

_____

_____

_____

_____

_____

_____

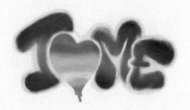

_____

_____

_____

_____

_____

_____

_____

_____

_____

_____

_____

_____

_____

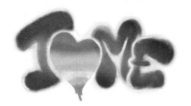

_____

_____

_____

_____

_____

_____

_____

_____

_____

_____

_____

_____

_____

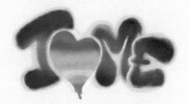

_____

_____

_____

_____

_____

_____

_____

_____

_____

_____

_____

_____

_____

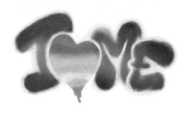

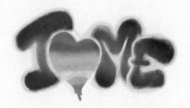

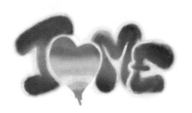

_____

_____

_____

_____

_____

_____

_____

_____

_____

_____

_____

_____

_____

_____

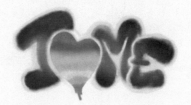

_____

_____

_____

_____

_____

_____

_____

_____

_____

_____

_____

_____

_____

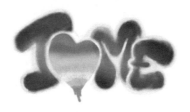

_____

_____

_____

_____

_____

_____

_____

_____

_____

_____

_____

_____

_____

_____

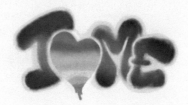

_____

_____

_____

_____

_____

_____

_____

_____

_____

_____

_____

_____

_____

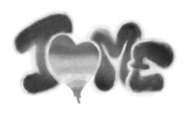

_____

_____

_____

_____

_____

_____

_____

_____

_____

_____

_____

_____

_____

_____

_____

_____

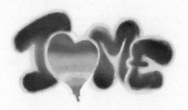

_____

_____

_____

_____

_____

_____

_____

_____

_____

_____

_____

_____

_____

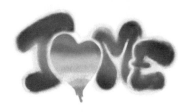

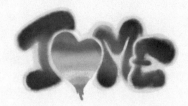

_____

_____

_____

_____

_____

_____

_____

_____

_____

_____

_____

_____

_____

_____

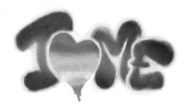

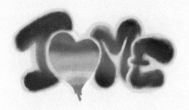

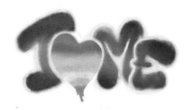

_____

_____

_____

_____

_____

_____

_____

_____

_____

_____

_____

_____

_____

_____

_____

_____

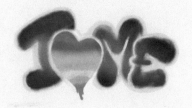

_____

_____

_____

_____

_____

_____

_____

_____

_____

_____

_____

_____

_____

_____

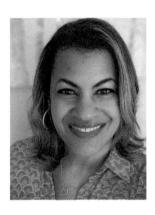

About the Author

Dr. Lisa Montgomery is a mom and wellness consultant who has learned how to manage her ongoing symptoms after surviving COVID-19. Along with crafting ways to improve her life, helping her daughter deal with mental health issues has made the mental health of our children a passionate pursuit.

With strength, perseverance, daily journaling and a grateful mindset, her daughter now has the tools to manage her life. Her journey inspired Dr. Lisa to create this story journal and base it on the universal symbol for hope – the rainbow. Dr. Lisa and her daughter share their message that there is always a helping hand and hope for healing.

Other Books
Riding the Rainbow: A short story and guided journal for kids

For more information, check out her website:

Made in the USA
Columbia, SC
09 July 2024

38306136R00060